NAVIGATING CLL WITH CONFIDENCE AND CARE

Mastering The Journey And Empowering Strategies For Confronting Chronic Lymphocytic Leukemia Disease For Vibrant Health

DR. WESLEY IAN

DISCLAIMER

The information in this book is not meant to replace professional medical advice, diagnosis, or treatment; rather, it is meant mainly for general informational reasons. If you have any questions about a medical problem, you should always consult your doctor or another trained health expert. Don't ever discount expert medical advice or put off getting it because of something you've read in this book.

Any negative effects or repercussions arising from the usage of the material provided herein are not the responsibility of the book's author or publisher. It should be noted by readers that the material in this book is not all-inclusive and might not address every facet of the subject. Furthermore, new research may have an impact on how health concerns are understood or treated because medical knowledge is always changing.

No particular test, treatment, method, or product mentioned in this book is endorsed or promoted by the author or publisher. The reader assumes all risk associated with using the information included in this book.

Before making any big decisions regarding your health, it's crucial to speak with a licensed healthcare provider. The relationship between a patient and their healthcare practitioner should not be replaced by this book, nor is it meant to offer medical advice.

The opinions presented in this book are the author's and may not necessarily represent those of the publisher. Any errors, omissions, or inaccuracies in the information in this book are not the responsibility of the author or publisher.

It is recommended that readers independently confirm any information contained in this book and speak with a healthcare provider about their specific medical needs and state of health.

TABLE OF CONTENTS

ABOUT THE BOOK

For those with Chronic Lymphocytic Leukemia (CLL) and those who care for them, "Navigating Chronic Lymphocytic Leukemia with Confidence and Care" is an extensive manual that is a great resource. An informative introduction to the book sets the stage for understanding CLL, its causes, and risk factors. With its comprehensive coverage of CLL diagnosis and staging, it gives readers a strong basis for understanding the complexity of this hematologic cancer.

The book discusses the practical and emotional difficulties of accepting a diagnosis of CLL. It looks at the emotional toll, how to communicate with family and friends effectively, and how crucial it is to get help when you need it during this trying time. This compassionate approach is essential for helping people deal with the emotional fallout after a CLL diagnosis, as it builds coping mechanisms and resilience.

Building a foundation of knowledge is the focus of the following chapters, which also provide an overview of CLL treatments, including immunotherapy, chemotherapy, watch and wait, and targeted therapies. The book walks readers through the process of making decisions by highlighting the need to comprehend treatment objectives, get second opinions, and consider taking part in clinical trials. People with CLL are better equipped to make decisions about their course of therapy after reading this section.

An important chapter titled "Living Well with CLL" discusses lifestyle modifications, such as exercise, diet, and methods for handling fatigue and mental health. Through the provision of useful guidance and insights, the book assists patients in maximizing their quality of life during CLL therapy.

"Care and Monitoring" and "Relationships and Support Systems" are essential since they address the continuous aspects of having CLL. They help readers stay proactive about their healthcare by guiding them through routine check-ups, monitoring, and managing side effects. The book also provides insightful advice on how to maintain a healthy balance between independence and reliance, communicate with friends and family, and create a strong support system.

The "Future Perspectives," gives it a forward-looking perspective. It looks at CLL research and developments, illuminating new therapies as well as the importance of patient involvement and advocacy. This book's forward-thinking strategy presents it as a dynamic, ever-evolving resource that gives readers a sense of empowerment and optimism for the future.

"Navigating Chronic Lymphocytic Leukemia with Confidence and Care" is essentially a source of information and encouragement that blends medical knowledge with compassionate direction. The book is an invaluable resource for people with CLL and those who care for them, as it covers all the facets of living with the disease, from the moment of diagnosis to the outlook for the future.

CHAPTER ONE

THE INTRODUCTION TO CLL

AN EXPLANATION OF CLL, OR CHRONIC LYMPHOCYTIC LEUKEMIA

As a well-known and complex hematologic cancer, chronic lymphocytic leukemia (CLL) requires a thorough understanding from both medical experts and the general public. This leukemia has significant clinical significance since it primarily affects the elderly population and is defined by the aberrant proliferation of mature cells. With a focus on risk factors, underlying causes, definition, and diagnostic procedures related to staging the disease to determine its severity, this introduction seeks to explore the complexities of CLL.

CLL: WHAT IS IT?

One kind of leukemia that is included in the larger group of hematological malignancies is CLL. The clonal growth of aberrant B-lymphocytes, mostly mature-looking cells, in the bone marrow, blood, and lymphatic tissues is what distinguishes this particular subtype. In contrast to acute leukemia, chronic lymphoblastic leukemia (CLL) usually advances slowly, with the aberrant cells building up over time. The immune system's capacity to successfully fight infections is compromised by the overproduction of these lymphocytes, which interferes with normal blood cell production and function. Deciphering the cellular and molecular pathways that underlie CLL is essential to understanding the disease's complexity.

REASONS AND DANGER FACTORS

It takes a complex effort to identify the causes and risk factors of CLL. Although the precise cause of CLL is still unknown, several factors have a role in its development. A major contributing factor is genetic predisposition; people with a family history of CLL are more susceptible. Furthermore, CLL has been connected to several chromosomal anomalies, including the deletion of certain genes. The risk profile is also influenced by environmental variables, such as radiation and exposure to specific chemicals.

To precisely understand the mechanisms behind the onset and progression of CLL, more research is needed due to the complex interactions between genetic and environmental variables.

IDENTIFICATION AND STAGE

For CLL to be properly managed, an accurate and fast diagnosis is essential. Blood tests, imaging studies, and clinical examinations are frequently used in conjunction with diagnosis. Finding distinctive markers on the surface of B-lymphocytes, such as CD5, CD19, and CD23, is essential for the diagnosis of CLL. For this, flow cytometry, a method that examines the properties of individual cells, is frequently used. To confirm the diagnosis and determine the degree of involvement, a bone marrow biopsy may also be carried out.

For CLL patients, staging plays a critical role in establishing their prognosis and directing their course of treatment. Based on the degree of lymphocyte infiltration and the existence of particular symptoms, two popular methods for classifying CLL into distinct stages are the Rai staging system and the Binet staging system. These staging systems give medical practitioners a framework for adjusting treatment plans based on the disease's severity.

Learning about CLL requires a thorough comprehension of its definition, underlying causes, risk factors, and complex diagnostic and staging procedures. This information serves as the cornerstone for developing therapeutic strategies that work and improve the general care of patients dealing with this complicated and long-term type of leukemia.

CHAPTER TWO

ACKNOWLEDGING CLL

MANAGING THE FIRST DIAGNOSIS

For patients and their loved ones, accepting a diagnosis of chronic lymphocytic leukemia (CLL) can be a difficult and upsetting process. An important part of this journey, one that is characterized by a variety of emotions and anxieties, is coping with the initial diagnosis. It frequently entails sifting through a deluge of information, comprehending the diagnosis' ramifications, and accepting that one will always have a chronic illness.

EFFECT ON EMOTIONS

A CLL diagnosis has a deep and individual emotional impact on each person. Common first feelings when the realization dawns that life may be drastically changed include shock, fear, and anxiety. An emotional rollercoaster might be exacerbated by future uncertainty and worries about the results of treatment.

Coping strategies differ greatly; some people find comfort in self-analysis and introspection, while others seek consolation from friends, family, or support organizations.

SPEAKING WITH CLOSE RELATIVES

Getting in touch with family and friends becomes essential to accepting a CLL diagnosis. It might be difficult to break the news to those you care about when you're struggling with your feelings and trying to explain complicated medical information. It is essential to have open and sincere communication to create a space where people feel free to voice their problems, ask questions, and receive emotional support. Family members frequently have a significant impact on giving the emotional support required for people to overcome upcoming obstacles.

LOOKING FOR ASSISTANCE

One of the most important steps in accepting CLL is to look for support. Having a network of sympathetic people, whether from medical professionals, support organizations, or counseling services, can greatly lessen the emotional strain. Both in-person and virtual support groups provide a forum for people to talk about their experiences, and trade knowledge, and find comfort in the common experience of living with chronic lymphoblastic leukemia. A secure environment for processing feelings and creating coping mechanisms specific to the difficulties presented by a chronic illness can be found in professional counseling.

Adjusting to the diagnosis of CLL is a complex process that entails managing the emotional fallout, talking to loved ones, and actively seeking out help. Accepting these facets of the journey might enable people to confront the difficulties presented by CLL with fortitude and a feeling of camaraderie, ultimately leading to a more comprehensive strategy for handling the intricacies of managing a chronic illness.

CHAPTER THREE

CREATING A BASIS OF KNOWLEDGE

AN OVERVIEW OF TREATMENTS FOR CLL

The main feature of chronic lymphocytic leukemia (CLL), a malignancy of the bone marrow and blood, is the slow build-up of aberrant white blood cells. Over time, the landscape of CLL treatment has changed dramatically, providing a variety of therapeutic alternatives catered to individual patient needs. Comprehending various therapeutic approaches is essential to developing a thorough understanding base.

APPROACH, WATCH, AND WAIT

One unique tactic that's frequently used in CLL management is the "Watch and Wait" approach. In contrast to many other malignancies, CLL can grow slowly, and not every patient needs treatment right once. Under the watch-and-wait strategy, medical professionals keep a careful eye on the patient's health through routine examinations and blood work before starting active therapy until there is proof of the disease progressing. When the condition is stable, this cautious observation helps to preserve quality of life and prevents needless procedures.

CHEMOTHERAPY

Chemotherapy has long been a mainstay of cancer treatment; in CLL, it is used to kill cancer cells that divide quickly. Traditional chemotherapy drugs, however, can have serious adverse effects that affect both healthy and malignant cells. Chemotherapy is often saved for CLL patients whose disease has progressed or who have not responded to other forms of treatment.

IMMUNOTHERAPY

By using the body's immune system to target and eliminate cancer cells, immunotherapy represents a paradigm leap in the treatment of cancer. Monoclonal antibodies are frequently utilized in immunotherapy for CLL. These antibodies can specifically identify and attach to CLL cells, designating them for immune system destruction or causing cell death directly. When compared to conventional chemotherapy, immunotherapy is frequently more tolerable and has fewer adverse effects.

SPECIALIZED TREATMENTS

A very promising new approach to treating CLL is targeted therapy, which targets particular chemicals essential to the development and viability of cancer cells. This class of drugs includes those that block signaling pathways essential for the survival of CLL cells, such as PI3K and BTK inhibitors. Compared to conventional chemotherapy, targeted therapies provide a more focused and targeted approach, which frequently leads to increased efficacy and fewer adverse effects.

There are several treatment options available for patients with chronic lymphocytic leukemia, each customized to the patient's unique needs and the unique features of the illness. In situations with indolent CLL, the watch-and-wait method permits meticulous surveillance; choices for more aggressive management include chemotherapy, immunotherapy, and targeted treatments. Ongoing developments in CLL therapies highlight how crucial it is for the field of oncology to have a dynamic and ever-evolving body of knowledge.

CHAPTER FOUR

CHOOSING THE RIGHT TREATMENT

MAKING TREATMENT DECISIONS

A crucial part of the healthcare process is figuring out treatment alternatives, which calls for cooperation between patients and medical staff. Making decisions about a patient's course of therapy entails carefully weighing the pros and disadvantages of each choice while taking into account the condition's specifics, the patient's characteristics, and possible hazards. Patients who are empowered to actively choose the best course of action based on their beliefs and preferences are the beneficiaries of informed decision-making.

COMPREHENDING THE OBJECTIVES OF TREATMENT

Patients and healthcare professionals must be both aware of the aims of treatment to make well-informed care decisions. Depending on the particular medical condition, these objectives could be anything from symptom relief and disease management to curative interventions. To match treatment objectives with each patient's unique preferences and values, open communication between patients and healthcare providers is crucial. Having a mutual understanding of the intended therapy goals is facilitated by setting reasonable expectations and talking about possible results.

SECOND VIEWS

When making treatment decisions, getting a second opinion is a useful and frequently advised step. It gives patients the chance to learn more from a different medical expert, resulting in a more thorough comprehension of their diagnosis and available treatments. Second views can provide comfort, validate the original diagnosis, or present other viewpoints that might result in different treatment philosophies. Maintaining a transparent and cooperative relationship with the primary healthcare team requires having open and honest conversations regarding the decision to seek a second opinion.

CLINICAL EXAMINATIONS

Clinical trials are essential for expanding our understanding of medicine and available treatments. When new solutions are being researched or when established treatments are failing, clinical trial participation may be taken into consideration. To help patients make an educated decision about potentially participating, healthcare practitioners might provide information about current clinical trials that are pertinent to the patient's condition.

Clinical trials present the possibility of gaining access to cutting-edge medicines and advancing medical knowledge, but they also entail inherent dangers and uncertainty. To make sure that their decision to participate in a clinical trial is in line with their objectives and values, patients should be fully educated about the trial's purpose, methods, potential benefits, and potential hazards.

Selecting a course of therapy necessitates a careful and cooperative approach that includes defining treatment objectives, getting second opinions, making treatment decisions, and thinking about taking part in clinical trials. Patients are empowered to make decisions that are in line with their own needs and values when there is open communication, collaborative decision-making, and a thorough examination of all available possibilities.

CHAPTER FIVE

GETTING BY WITH CLL

MODIFICATIONS TO LIFESTYLE

A healthy lifestyle is important for people with Chronic Lymphocytic Leukemia (CLL) since it promotes general health and well-being. Finding a balance between preserving a sense of normalcy and adjusting to any unique requirements that CLL may impose is crucial. This can involve making adjustments to social events, job schedules, and everyday routines. Providing a welcoming atmosphere that takes into account the difficulties posed by CLL can make it easier for people to go about their everyday lives.

EXERCISE AND DIET

When it comes to maintaining the general health of people with CLL, nutrition is vital. A balanced diet can assist the body's ability to withstand the effects of the disease and its therapies, maintain energy levels, and strengthen the immune system.

To promote total nutritional wellness, include a range of fruits, vegetables, lean proteins, and whole grains. Exercise regularly can also be quite helpful in treating CLL. Engaging in physical activity not only aids in maintaining a healthy weight but also improves mood, energy levels, and general well-being.

HANDLING EXHAUSTION

For those with CLL, fatigue is a prevalent problem that is frequently brought on by the illness or its therapies. A mix of dietary modifications, lifestyle alterations, and deliberate energy conservation are necessary for managing fatigue effectively.

Putting things in order of importance, taking regular pauses, and sticking to a sleep schedule will all help prevent drowsiness? People with CLL must pay attention to their bodies, let medical professionals know what they need, and ask friends and family for help to cope with the effects of exhaustion daily.

EMOTIONAL HEALTH

Living well with CLL requires maintaining one's emotional health because the condition and its therapies can have a significant negative effect on mental health. To manage the psychological effects of chronic lymphoblastic disease (CLL), it's important to establish a solid support system, communicate candidly with medical professionals, and, if necessary, seek out support groups or professional counseling. Developing coping skills through artistic expression, mindfulness, or meditation can also help build emotional resilience. A vital component of the comprehensive approach to well-being for those with CLL is recognizing and treating the emotional elements of the illness.

A comprehensive approach that includes lifestyle modifications, appropriate nutrition, consistent exercise, efficient fatigue management, and attention to mental well-being is necessary to live well with CLL.

CHAPTER SIX

HANDLING AND OBSERVATION

FREQUENT INSPECTIONS AND SURVEILLANCE

Frequent monitoring and check-ups are essential for preserving general health and averting possible medical problems. These annual physicals, which are usually planned on the recommendation of medical specialists, enable people to take proactive measures to address any new health issues. The body mass index (BMI), general organ function, and vital signs are among the physical well-being factors that healthcare professionals evaluate during these examinations. Frequent monitoring offers the chance to identify possible health problems early on, facilitating prompt intervention and preventive measures.

IMAGING AND BLOOD TESTS

A person's health state can be ascertained by basic diagnostic procedures such as blood tests and imaging investigations. Blood tests examine several indicators, including blood sugar, liver function, and cholesterol levels, and they provide important details on how the body is internally working. Imaging methods provide detailed representations of internal structures and help identify abnormalities, cancers, and other anomalies. Examples of these methods include X-rays, CT scans, and MRIs. These diagnostic techniques play a crucial role in helping medical professionals make precise diagnoses and thoughtful treatment recommendations.

CONTROLLING ADVERSE REACTIONS

Controlling side effects is a critical component of care, especially for patients receiving medical interventions or treatments. Adverse effects from medications and therapies can range in severity from a little discomfort to more serious reactions. Addressing and reducing these adverse effects requires effective communication with healthcare practitioners. To enable timely modifications to treatment plans, patients should be proactive in reporting any symptoms or concerns to their healthcare team. The implementation of a collaborative strategy guarantees the efficient management of side effects, hence improving the overall quality of care and treatment outcomes.

COLLABORATING WITH HEALTHCARE PROVIDERS

Effective monitoring and care require strong collaboration with healthcare practitioners. Facilitating transparent channels of communication cultivates a cooperative partnership between patients and their medical teams. Individuals can address concerns, talk about any changes in their health, and get advice on managing chronic diseases during routine appointments. Patients should actively communicate with their healthcare providers, providing details about their symptoms, way of life, and compliance with recommended course of action. This collaboration improves treatment efficacy, advances a thorough comprehension of medical issues, and enables collaborative decision-making during treatment.

A comprehensive approach to healthcare must include the ideas of routine examinations and monitoring, blood testing and imaging, managing side effects, and collaborating with medical professionals. These procedures aid in the correct diagnosis of illnesses, the timely identification of possible health problems, and the efficient administration of medical interventions. People can maximize their well-being and develop cooperative relationships with healthcare providers by actively engaging in their care, which guarantees a proactive and knowledgeable approach to sustaining health.

CHAPTER SEVEN

CONNECTIONS AND SAFETY NETS

SPEAKING WITH LOVED ONES AND FRIENDS

The foundation of wholesome relationships with family and friends is effective communication. Honest and transparent communication promotes empathy, trust, and understanding. Sharing one's ideas and feelings with close ones during happy or difficult times creates a support network that can offer consolation and direction. But good communication is more than simply self-expression; it also entails empathy and attentive listening. Being sensitive to the wants and needs of friends and family lays the groundwork for deep connections that strengthen the ties that keep relationships going throughout time.

Any partnership will inevitably include handling disagreements. To keep miscommunication from getting worse at these moments, clear communication becomes essential. Establishing common ground, making concessions, and honoring one another's viewpoints are all components of healthy communication. Friends and family relationships become a source of strength and enhance general well-being when they are acknowledged and respected.

MAINTAINING EQUILIBRIUM DEPENDENCY AND INDEPENDENCE

In any relationship, striking a healthy balance between reliance and independence requires careful dancing moves. Autonomy is necessary for personal development and self-discovery, but interdependence is just as important for creating a solid support network. Finding this balance requires encouraging a sense of shared accountability and mutual reliance while also acknowledging and respecting each person's boundaries.

Respecting one's personality, hobbies, and aspirations is essential to preserving independence in a partnership. It necessitates candid discussion of personal needs and goals. Constructing a safe environment where people can rely on one another for companionship, support, and emotional assistance is another aspect of developing dependence. Both the relationship and the individuals can grow as a result of this balance.

It is important to realize that interdependence does not mean weakness. It denotes a sound reliance on one another's advantages, fostering a symbiotic connection in which both sides advance the prosperity and development of the alliance.

CREATING A NETWORK OF SUPPORT

A strong support system is essential to emotional health. It includes a wide range of people who provide various viewpoints and ways of support, going beyond close friends and family. It takes deliberate labor and commitment in relationships across a range of life arenas to build such a network.

In a support system, variety is essential. Colleagues or mentors can offer professional direction, while family and close friends can offer emotional support. Participating in social or community groups increases network size by providing a feeling of community and common interests. The advent of digital technology has additionally broadened the scope for global connections with like-minded people, underscoring the significance of a diverse network of support.

One essential component of a support system is reciprocity. Developing deep relationships requires being able to support others when they need it. The ties within the network are strengthened and a sense of community is fostered by this mutual aid.

The cornerstone ideas for establishing and maintaining good relationships are clear communication, a balanced perspective on independence and dependency, and the deliberate development of a wide range of support systems. The whole richness of one's social network, emotional fortitude, and personal well-being are all greatly enhanced by these factors.

CHAPTER EIGHT

PROSPECTS FOR THE FUTURE

DEVELOPMENTS IN CHRONIC LYMPHOCYTIC LEUKEMIA (CLL) RESEARCH AND PRACTICE

Over the past few years, the field of Chronic Lymphocytic Leukemia (CLL) research has witnessed significant strides, marking a pivotal era in our understanding of the disease and its underlying mechanisms. The advent of advanced technologies, such as next-generation sequencing, has facilitated the identification of novel genetic mutations associated with CLL, shedding light on the intricate molecular landscape of the disease. Researchers have delved into the intricate interplay between genetic and environmental factors, unraveling the complexities that govern CLL's development and progression.

Moreover, the exploration of novel biomarkers has emerged as a cornerstone in CLL research, enabling more precise diagnosis, prognostication, and personalized treatment approaches. The identification of specific molecular markers has paved the way for a more nuanced understanding of CLL heterogeneity, offering the potential to tailor therapies based on individual patient profiles. As research in CLL continues to progress, the integration of multi-omics data and comprehensive analyses holds promise for uncovering additional layers of complexity, ultimately contributing to more effective and targeted therapeutic strategies.

EMERGING TREATMENTS FOR CLL

The landscape of CLL treatment has undergone a transformative evolution with the emergence of novel therapeutic modalities. One of the notable breakthroughs is the advent of targeted therapies, such as BTK inhibitors and BCL-2 inhibitors, which have demonstrated remarkable efficacy in managing CLL. These agents, designed to selectively target specific pathways implicated in CLL pathogenesis, have showcased unprecedented clinical responses, offering improved outcomes and enhanced tolerability compared to traditional chemotherapy.

Immunotherapy has also emerged as a promising avenue in CLL treatment, with the development of chimeric antigen receptor (CAR) T-cell therapy. This innovative approach involves reprogramming a patient's T cells to recognize and eliminate CLL cells, representing a paradigm shift in the treatment landscape. Ongoing research is focused on refining CAR T-cell therapy, addressing challenges such as durability of response and managing potential side effects, to optimize its clinical applicability.

Furthermore, the exploration of combination therapies, leveraging the synergistic effects of different agents, is a key focus in current CLL research. Clinical trials investigating the efficacy and safety of various combinations aim to establish new standards of care, to achieve deeper and more durable responses, particularly in the context of relapsed or refractory disease.

PATIENT ADVOCACY AND INVOLVEMENT IN CLL:

In parallel with advancements in CLL research and treatment, the role of patient advocacy and involvement has gained prominence in shaping the landscape of CLL care. Recognizing the importance of patient perspectives, advocacy groups, and organizations have played a pivotal role in amplifying patient voices, fostering awareness, and advocating for improved access to innovative therapies.

Patients and their advocates have become active participants in the decision-making process, contributing to discussions on treatment options, clinical trial design, and healthcare policy. This collaborative approach not only empowers patients but also enriches the healthcare ecosystem by incorporating diverse perspectives into the development and evaluation of CLL therapies.

Furthermore, patient advocacy initiatives have been instrumental in destigmatizing CLL and raising public awareness about the disease. By fostering a sense of community and support, these efforts contribute to a more comprehensive understanding of the psychosocial aspects of living with CLL, addressing the holistic needs of patients beyond medical treatment.

As we navigate the future of CLL research and care, the synergy between scientific advancements, innovative treatments, and patient advocacy is poised to shape a more patient-centric and effective paradigm for managing this complex hematologic malignancy.